Eating Right

SIGNAL HI

■■■K:

PUBLICATIO

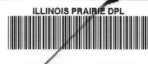

This book was produced in
collaboration with the
**American Institute for
Preventive Medicine.**

1997 printing
Copyright © 1994
New Readers Press
Publishing Division of Laubach Literacy International
Box 131, Syracuse, New York 13210-0131

Printed in the United States of America

Information graphics by Shane Kelley
Illustrations by Richard Ewing
Icons by Melanie White
Cover photo: DAVE REVETTE

9 8 7 6 5 4 3 2 1

Library of Congress Cataloging-in-Publication Data
Eating right.
p. cm.
"Produced in collaboration with the American Institute
for Preventive Medicine" -- T. p. verso.
ISBN 1-56420-021-3
1. Nutrition. 2. Readers (adult) I. New Readers Press.
II. American Institute for Preventive Medicine.
RA784.E165   1993
613.2--dc20   93-34108
                                        CIP

Contents

Preface

Information is power.

Being informed means being able to make choices. When you can make choices, you are not helpless. Having information is the first step toward being in control of a situation. It is a way to get more out of life.

This book, *Eating Right,* discusses issues that affect everyone—diet and nutrition. It gives useful information and suggestions for making good food choices.

The books in the For Your Information series are developed with experts from lead agencies in each topic area. This book was developed with help from the American Institute for Preventive Medicine (AIPM). AIPM develops and provides wellness programs and publications. It is based in Farmington Hills, Michigan.

Thanks to the following people for their contribution to the content of *Eating Right:* Don R. Powell, Ph.D., founder and president of AIPM; Elaine Frank, M.Ed., R.D., vice president of AIPM; Annette B. Natow, Ph.D., R.D., of Nutrition Consultants; and Jo-Ann Heslin, M.A., R.D., of Nutrition Consultants.

And special thanks to Cynthia Moritz for her writing.

In this book

- Words in **bold** are explained in the glossary on pages 91–95.
- People may be referred to either as "he" or "she."
- At the end of some chapters, you'll find resources for help or for more information.

Introduction

Most people like to eat. Many people worry that what they like to eat is not good for them, though. Many people would like to improve their diets. They may not be able to for a few reasons:

- They do not know enough about good **nutrition**—the foods they eat.
- They are afraid they will have to give up all the foods they love.
- They think a healthy diet will be too hard to follow.
- They think a healthy diet will cost too much.

Good nutrition is important. If you live to be 70 years old, you will probably eat more than 75,000 meals. Giving your body the fuel it needs in those meals may help you reach age 70 with a healthy body and mind.

If the meals you eat do not give your body what it needs, it may affect your health. Poor nutrition increases your chances of getting many diseases. They include **heart disease, high blood pressure, diabetes,** and **osteoporosis** (a bone-thinning disease). Poor nutrition also cuts down on your energy.

No one can promise that if you have a healthy diet, you will not get any of these diseases. Your health is affected by other factors, too. They include:

- what kinds of diseases people in your family have had
- how much exercise you get
- how much stress you have in your life

A good diet can increase your chances of staying healthy. If you do get sick, a healthy diet makes your body more able to fight the illness.

Eating a healthy diet is not hard to do. You do not always have to give up the foods you love. A healthy diet does not need to be hard to follow. It does not have to cost a lot, either.

This book tells you about **nutrients.** Nutrients are materials that your body gets from food. They are the building blocks of your body and the fuel it uses. You can find out in this book how to include them in your diet.

The book shows you some easy ways to improve your diet. It suggests ways to shop wisely—to save money and eat healthy at the same time. It also describes how to handle food safely.

This book can help you learn how to make good food choices when you are eating out. It gives ideas for how to lose weight in a healthy way and keep from gaining it back.

At the end of some chapters is a list of places to find out more information.

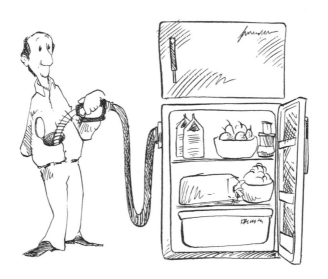

General Rules for Good Nutrition

- Eat many kinds of foods. This way you get many different nutrients.
- Do not eat too much of any one food. No food is good if you eat too much of it.
- Change your eating habits slowly. You are more likely to stick with a new way of eating if you make only a few changes at a time.

Life Stories

Here are some examples of people who want to improve their diets. They are not sure how. Imagine they are reading this book, too. At the end, you will see how they have decided to change their diets.

Andrea and Mike

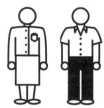 Andrea, 24, and Mike, 29, are a married couple. They both have jobs, and often do not get home until six or seven o'clock. Neither of them likes to cook. At home, they often eat canned soups, frozen dinners, or take-out food.

Breakfast is usually coffee and a donut. Mike sometimes skips lunch. When he does eat lunch, it is often a hot dog or a grilled cheese sandwich, with a soda. He buys them from the truck that comes to his work site. Andrea has a salad or a sandwich at her company's cafeteria.

Mike's doctor has told him that he is a little overweight. His **cholesterol** is rather high.

The couple would like to have a baby soon. Andrea knows she should improve her diet before—and while—she is pregnant.

Sonya

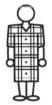 Sonya is a single mother. Each of Sonya's three daughters has her own favorite foods. It seems to Sonya that no two of them will eat the same thing. She spends a lot of time getting the girls to eat. She does not spend so much time making sure their diets are healthy.

The dentist has said that Sonya's middle daughter has too much **tooth decay**. She should not eat a lot of sugar. All the girls like food with a lot of sugar.

Sonya would also like to spend less money on groceries. As a single parent, she has trouble making ends meet. Going to the grocery store is difficult, too. She's always in a rush, and the girls are always begging for candy.

Karl

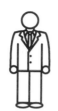 Karl, 52, is a salesperson. Karl has just been told he has high blood pressure. His doctor says he should lose from 20 to 30 pounds. He should also cut out most of the salt in his diet. This will be hard. Karl eats a diet that is high in fat and salt. His sales job requires him to eat out a lot. Most menus are full of fatty foods. Karl loves them.

When he is home, Karl eats mostly canned fruits and vegetables. He fries most meat and uses a lot of butter on bread and vegetables.

To find out more

After you read this book, you may want more information on nutrition. Call:

The American Dietetic Association
(800) 366-1655
This is a nutrition hotline.

Chapter 1
Nutrients

Your body is made up of billions of tiny cells. To work properly, each cell needs materials from the food you eat. These materials are called nutrients. There are about 40 nutrients. They fall into six groups:

1. water
2. protein
3. carbohydrates
4. fats
5. minerals
6. vitamins

The chart on pages 14–15 lists the nutrients and their benefits. It also gives common sources of each nutrient.

Nutrient	What it does
water	• gets rid of waste • carries nutrients through the body
protein 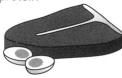	• needed for growth and repairing the body • gives you energy
carbohydrates 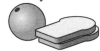	• give you energy • provide fiber • provide vitamins and minerals
fats 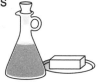	• give you energy • carry some vitamins through the body • keep the body warm
minerals 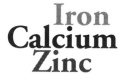 Iron Calcium Zinc	• keep bones and teeth strong • help nerves and muscles work • help prevent sickness • help make healthy blood
vitamins 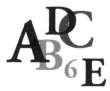 A D C B 6 E	• help prevent sickness • help the body use other nutrients • keep the body looking and feeling good • help form bones, muscles, and teeth

Some places to get it	Tips
• liquids (water, juices, milk)	Try to drink 6−8 glasses of water a day.
• meat, chicken, and fish • dried beans • nuts • eggs and dairy products	Eat some protein every day.
• grains and cereals • dried beans, pasta • fruits and vegetables	Eat more whole-grain breads and cereals.
• butter and margarine • other oils • nuts • animal products	A little fat goes a long way.
• dairy products • vegetables and fresh fruits • dried fruits • meat, chicken, and fish • tofu	A balanced diet provides all the minerals you need.
• vegetables and fruits • grains and cereals • meat, chicken, and fish • dairy products (milk, cheese, yogurt)	Eat a variety of foods. Try to eat 5 fruits or vegetables every day.

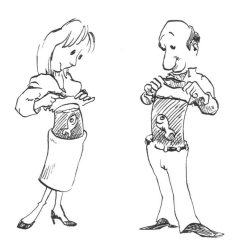

Water

Believe it or not, your body contains more water than anything else. Women are made up of about 60 percent water. For men it is about 70 percent. Water is the most important nutrient. Each cell in your body needs it. You would die a lot sooner from lack of water than from lack of food.

Water carries other nutrients through the body. It also removes waste from the cells. The body gets rid of waste through the water in sweat and urine.

Some of the water in your body comes from the foods you eat. Some comes from the liquids you drink. Most adults should drink from six to eight glasses of water each day.

Protein

Some of protein's many jobs are:

- forming new **tissues** and replacing old
- helping nutrients travel to and from the body's cells
- helping the blood to clot
- helping to fight diseases

Your body stores very little protein. So you should eat some protein every day. This is not usually a problem in the United States. Most of us eat at least twice as much protein as we need.

Protein is contained in foods that come from both animals and plants. Animal proteins are more complete. That means the body can use them easily.

Vegetable proteins are not as complete. You can make vegetable protein more complete by eating more than one kind at the same meal. Some good combinations are corn and beans, or peanut butter and whole-wheat bread.

Another way to make vegetable protein more complete is to eat it with a small amount of animal protein.

Carbohydrates

There are two types of carbohydrates:

- **complex carbohydrates,** also called starches. They are in fruits, vegetables, and grain products.
- **simple carbohydrates,** or sugars. They are in jelly, syrups, fruits, and vegetables.

Most Americans get most of their sugar from treats such as candy, ice cream, and cookies. These are sometimes called "empty calorie" foods. They give you a lot of **calories** but few nutrients.

Carbohydrates are the best source of energy. It is best to eat foods that are rich in complex carbohydrates. They are **digested** more slowly. Foods that contain them, like fruits and vegetables, also contain lots of other nutrients.

Complex carbohydrates also provide **fiber.** Fiber is not a nutrient. It is material that the body cannot break down. It passes through the body, helping the bowels to work properly. Experts tell us to eat more fiber for good health. Eating fiber may help prevent some types of cancer. The chart on page 19 lists some common sources of fiber.

Simple carbohydrates like sugar provide energy, but also a lot of calories.

Fiber source	Examples
beans 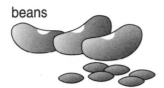	lima beans navy beans kidney beans lentils
fruit 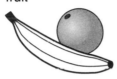	oranges bananas peaches
vegetables 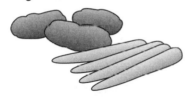	broccoli potatoes corn carrots peas
grains 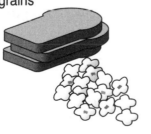	whole-grain bread brown rice shredded wheat cereal popcorn

Fats

There are two types of fat:

- **Body fat.** This is the fat on your body. If you eat more calories than you need, you will make too much body fat. That's not healthy. You need very little fat in your diet. Your body can make fat out of extra protein or carbohydrates.
- **Dietary fat.** This is fat that you eat. You should eat a small amount of fat. It helps your body to absorb some nutrients. Dietary fat comes from animal products such as meat, cheese, butter, and milk. Vegetable oils, salad dressing, and margarine also contain dietary fat.

Your body can use the fat you eat as energy. Fats supply more than twice the energy of carbohydrates or protein.

That may sound good. It is, however, one of the reasons that people gain too much weight. If you are eating high-fat foods, it is easy to eat more calories than you need and still not feel full.

For example, think of a high-fat food: one slice of apple pie, with a scoop of ice cream. That's not a lot, right? Yet, to consume the same number of calories in low-fat foods, you would have to eat:

- 7 apples or
- 30 carrots or
- 60 stalks of celery

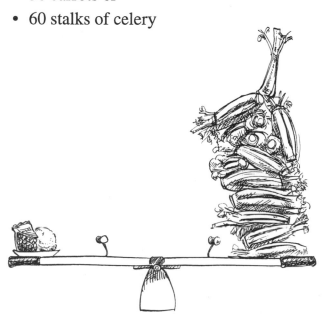

Minerals

Minerals make up only about four percent of your body weight. But they do some important jobs. Two of the important minerals are:

- **Calcium.** It helps to build bones and teeth and keep them strong. It helps cuts to stop bleeding.

  Many Americans do not get enough calcium in their diets. If you do not get enough calcium, your bones become thin. In children, this causes a disease called rickets. In adults, especially older women, it causes osteoporosis. Osteoporosis makes bones become thinner and weaker. They break more easily.

  Calcium is found in milk and other dairy foods. You can also get it from some vegetables, such as spinach, broccoli, and kale.

- **Iron.** It helps to make healthy blood. It helps oxygen get to the cells. Cells die without oxygen. Iron is found in red meat and fish. You can also get it from green leafy vegetables and dried fruits.

  If you do not get enough iron in your diet, you may develop **anemia.** Anemic people feel tired a lot. Their bodies have trouble fighting off infections.

  The chart on page 23 lists some common sources of calcium and iron.

Calcium sources	Iron sources
• milk, yogurt, cheese	• red meat
• other dairy products	• fish, shellfish
• sardines	• chicken
• salmon with the bones	• turkey liver
• clams	• kidney
• oysters	• enriched breads
• tofu	and cereals
• green leafy vegetables	• egg yolks
• broccoli	• green leafy vegetables
• kale	• dried fruits
• oranges	• blackstrap molasses
• tangerines	
• grapefruit	

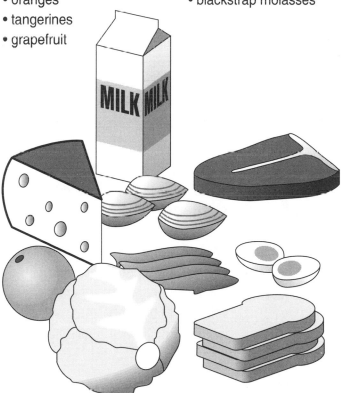

Vitamin	Food Source
A	liver, eggs, enriched milk and dairy products, dark green vegetables, deep yellow fruits like apricots, peaches, cantaloupe, carrots, sweet potatoes, pumpkin, squash
B1	meat (especially pork), liver, fish, green peas, beans, collard greens, oranges, asparagus, whole grains, wheat germ, nuts, yeast
B2	liver, kidneys, lean meat, chicken, tuna, sardines, milk and dairy products, eggs, dark green vegetables, whole grains, beans
B3	liver, lean meat, fish, chicken, turkey, milk, eggs, nuts, beans, dark green vegetables, whole grains
C	oranges, tangerines, grapefruit, strawberries, cantaloupe, brussels sprouts, broccoli, green peppers, collard greens, cauliflower, cabbage, tomatoes, asparagus

Vitamins

Your body needs 13 vitamins. They are:

* vitamin A
* vitamin D
* vitamin E
* vitamin K
* vitamin C
* thiamin
* riboflavin
* niacin
* vitamin B6
* vitamin B12
* folacin
* pantothenic acid
* biotin

Each vitamin has its own job. Vitamins help the body work properly. They also help the body use protein, carbohydrates, and fats. They help to form red blood cells.

Many different foods contain vitamins. If you are worried that you do not get all the vitamins you need from the foods you eat, you could take a **multivitamin** each day. If you eat a healthy diet, though, you will get all the vitamins you need. The chart on page 24 shows common food sources of five important vitamins.

Additives

Sometimes chemicals called additives are added to the food you buy in a store. This is done to:

- make the food look, taste, or feel better
- add nutrients that do not occur in the food naturally
- make the food last longer without going bad

Additives are in about 10 percent of the food you eat. More than 90 percent of the additives most people eat are the sugar and salt they add themselves.

Some people think you should avoid all food additives. This is not necessary. It is more important to eat as many fresh foods as you can. Try to limit high-fat, high-calorie foods that have few nutrients.

Chapter 2
Getting Good Nutrition

Experts keep learning more about how the food we eat affects our health. They know enough already to give us guidelines for a healthy diet. These are the basic guidelines:

1. Eat many types of foods.
2. Stay at a healthy weight.
3. Choose a diet low in fat and cholesterol.
4. Eat plenty of vegetables, fruits, and grains.
5. Limit sugar in your diet.
6. Limit salt (**sodium**) in your diet.
7. Limit alcohol in your diet.

If you follow these guidelines, you will probably get enough of the nutrients you need.

Eat many types of foods

Wouldn't it be nice if your doctor could tell you one food you should eat to keep healthy? As long as you got enough of this one food, you could eat anything else you wanted.

Of course, this is not possible. No one food has enough of all the nutrients we need. Think about calcium and iron. They are two nutrients you need. Milk gives you calcium, but little iron. Meat supplies iron, but not much calcium. No one food can give you enough of both.

Stay at a healthy weight

Both eating too much and eating too little can harm your health.

Being too fat is common in the U.S. It increases your chances of getting high blood pressure, heart disease, **stroke,** diabetes, and some types of cancer.

Being too thin is more rare. If you are a woman, it increases your chances of getting osteoporosis.

Your doctor can give you some idea of what is a healthy weight for you. These factors all make a difference:

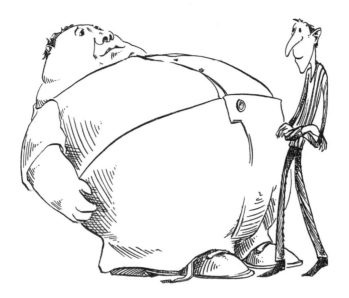

- your sex
- your age
- your height
- your build
- where the fat is located in your body. Fat around the belly is a greater health risk than fat in the hips or thighs.

Choose a diet low in fat and cholesterol

People who eat a lot of high-fat foods are more likely to be fat or get certain types of cancer. Eating lots of **saturated fat** and cholesterol increases your chances of getting heart disease.

Saturated fat comes mainly from animal fats such as butter or the fat on meat. Vegetable oils, except for coconut and palm oil, are a little better. They contain mostly **unsaturated fat.** Cholesterol is found in animal foods like meat, cheese, and eggs.

Fat contains more than twice the calories of carbohydrates or protein. That is why food experts advise getting no more than 30 percent of your calories from fat.

The amount of saturated fat in your diet should be no more than 10 percent of your calories.

The chart on page 31 gives tips on reducing fat in your diet.

Eat plenty of vegetables, fruits, and grains

These foods are usually low in fat. They contain lots of complex carbohydrates, **dietary fiber,** vitamins, and minerals.

Nutritionists advise that you eat at least this amount of each type of food each day:

- vegetables—three servings
- fruit—two servings
- grains—six servings. Grain products include breads, cereals, pasta, and rice.

Source of fat or cholesterol	Try instead
fried foods	steaming, boiling, or baking vegetables
	broiling, roasting, or baking meat on a rack so fat drains off
using butter and margarine for flavor	herbs and spices
salad dressing	lemon juice on salads
butter and shortening in baking	margarine or oil
whole milk	skim milk
sour cream and mayonnaise	plain lowfat yogurt
fatty cuts of meat	leaner cuts of meat; trim fat
egg yolks	using just the whites or more whites than yolks
chicken skin	removing skin before cooking

Limit sugar in your diet

Foods high in sugar have a lot of calories, but few nutrients. Most people should limit the amount of sugar in their diets.

What you put in your sugar bowl is not the only sugar you need to worry about. Some other common sugars are:

- honey
- brown sugar
- syrup
- molasses

Check the labels of foods you buy. Do they contain such things as corn syrup, fructose, maltose, and lactose? Those are different kinds of sugar, too.

Eating a lot of sugar can also cause your teeth to decay. Sugar is contained in many foods and drinks, such as cookies, ice cream, sodas, and some fruit drinks.

Limit salt (sodium) in your diet

Your body needs some sodium. Most people eat much more sodium than they need, however. Eating too much sodium increases your chances of having high blood pressure.

Table salt contains sodium. Some sodium in foods you buy is "hidden." Salt or sodium may

Where's the sugar?	Where's the sodium?
table sugar (sucrose)	table salt
brown sugar	onion salt
raw sugar	celery salt
glucose	garlic salt
fructose	meat tenderizer
maltose	bouillon
lactose	baking powder
honey	baking soda
syrup	monosodium glutamate
corn sweetener	soy sauce
high-fructose corn sweetener	steak sauce
molasses	barbecue sauce
	ketchup
	mustard
	Worcestershire sauce
	salad dressings
	pickles
	chili sauce
	relish

not be included on the list of ingredients. Any ingredient that has sodium, salt, or soda as part of its name contains sodium. Some examples are baking soda, onion salt, and monosodium glutamate. Soy sauce also contains a lot of sodium.

The chart on this page lists sources of salt and sugar. Look for them in **ingredient lists.**

Limit alcohol in your diet

Alcohol supplies calories, but few nutrients. It is linked with many health problems. Some people become **addicted** to alcohol.

Men who choose to drink need to limit themselves to two drinks per day. Women should drink even less alcohol, no more than one drink per day.

Some people should not drink alcohol at all. They include:

- women who are pregnant or trying to get pregnant
- people who plan to drive or operate machinery
- people who plan to do other things that require sharp attention
- people who are taking medication
- people who cannot limit their drinking
- children and teenagers

The Food Guide Pyramid

The **Food Guide Pyramid** on page 35 shows about how much you should have each day of foods from different groups. You should eat the most from the base of the pyramid.

Food Guide Pyramid

A guide to daily food choices

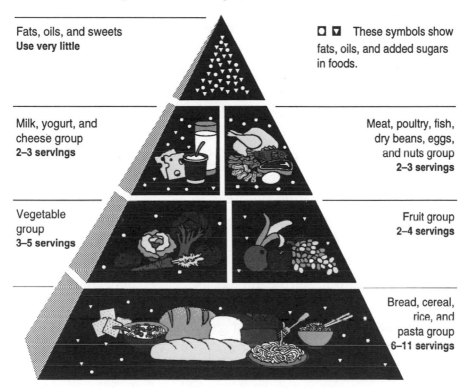

Fats, oils, and sweets
Use very little

◻ ▽ These symbols show fats, oils, and added sugars in foods.

Milk, yogurt, and cheese group
2–3 servings

Meat, poultry, fish, dry beans, eggs, and nuts group
2–3 servings

Vegetable group
3–5 servings

Fruit group
2–4 servings

Bread, cereal, rice, and pasta group
6–11 servings

The Food Guide Pyramid can help you eat a balanced diet. As you plan your meals, be sure to include items from each group. The Pyramid lists the number of servings from each group you should eat each day.

If you miss out on a certain group, you can always fill in with a snack. For example, if you've only had three fruits or vegetables, snack on an apple, or some carrot sticks.

All the food groups in the Pyramid are important. You need the least amount of fat and sugar, though.

SOURCE: U.S. Department of Agriculture/U.S. Department of Health and Human Resources

Healthy Vegetarian Diets

Some people choose not to eat meat. They are called **vegetarians.** There are many reasons why people choose to become vegetarians. Some believe it is wrong to eat animals. Others do it for health or religious reasons.

There are different kinds of vegetarian diets. Some vegetarians just cut out meat and fish. Others cut out eggs and dairy products, too.

A balanced vegetarian diet is as healthy as any diet. People do not need to eat meat to live. But everyone needs to be sure to get enough protein from the foods they eat. Vegetarians use plant proteins like beans to get enough protein.

Children can be raised as vegetarians. All babies must get enough protein, though. Otherwise, they may not grow as well as they should. This protein can come from breast milk, **infant formula, soy milk,** and other vegetable proteins. Check with your doctor to help you choose the best way.

To find out more

For more information about the seven nutrition guidelines, call:

The American Dietetic Association
(800) 366-1655
This is a nutrition hotline.

For more information on how diet affects disease, call:

American Cancer Society
(800) 227-2345

American Heart Association. Call the office listed in your phone book.

Cancer Information Service
(800) 422-6237

Chapter 3
Life Stages and Nutrition

The parents of a toddler worry. Their daughter ate a lot as a baby. Yet now she eats only a few bites at each meal. Some days she seems to live on air alone.

The father of a teenager is amazed. His son eats more than he does. He cannot believe the boy does not get fat.

These eating habits are normal. At different stages of life, the body has different food needs. The chart on pages 40–41 shows this. Most of this book is concerned with the food needs of young or middle-aged adults. This chapter is about the food needs of people at some other stages:

- babies
- small children
- older children
- teenagers
- older adults
- pregnant women

Babies

Until they are 4 to 6 months old, most babies need only breast milk. Breast milk has all of the nutrients that babies need. It also protects them against some diseases.

Some mothers have trouble nursing, or do not want to. Their babies can be fed infant formula instead. Babies can get the nutrients they need from formula.

Some parents start to feed their babies solid food when they are only a couple of months old. Babies that age do not need solid food. Their bodies cannot handle solid foods yet.

Babies are ready for solids sometime between the ages of 4 and 6 months. Doctors usually advise baby cereal as the baby's first food. It should be made with a single kind of grain, such as rice or oats. It should also contain extra iron.

Life Stages

Stage	Needs
babies (up to 6 months)	breast milk; infant formula
babies (6 months and up)	a single-grain cereal; add fruits and vegetables slowly
small children (up to 3 years)	need less, will eat less—don't worry as long as they stay healthy
older children (4–12 years)	serving size is 1 tablespoon for each year old (5 tablespoons for a 5-year-old)
teenagers	need a lot, will eat a lot; important to eat right foods; need a lot of nutrients
older people	need fewer calories, but the same nutrients; may gain weight, so need to keep active
pregnant/nursing women	should gain 24–35 pounds

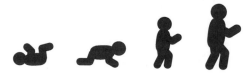

Servings per day			
Dairy	**Protein**	**Fruits/ Vegetables**	**Grains**
as much as needed			
as many as needed			
2	2	4+	4+
2–3	2–3	4+	4+
4	2–3	4+	4+
2	2–3	4+	4+
4	2–3	4+	4+

After the baby is used to eating cereal, parents should feed her strained fruits and vegetables. They should only give the baby one new food a week, if possible. If not, they should wait at least three days between food changes. Then, if the baby has a reaction to a food, they will know which food caused it.

Small children

For such little people, babies eat a lot. That is because they are growing quickly. Children start eating less once they become toddlers, however. Parents often feel that their small children do not eat enough.

Don't worry about it. It is natural for a small child to need less food. His growth has slowed down a lot.

Small children may not get all the nutrients they need in one meal. They may not get all their nutrients even in a whole day. That is all right. Their diets tend to balance out over a week or two.

So if your child wants only peanut butter one day, and only bananas the next, do not be too concerned. But don't let your child eat too much sugar or fat. If your child is eating healthy foods, he is probably getting the nutrients he needs.

Older children

Children need to eat enough to have energy for their daily activities. They also need to eat enough to grow. But you do not want your child to become fat.

Nutritionists say children should have each day:

- two to three servings of dairy products
- two servings of meat or other protein
- at least five servings of fruits and vegetables
- at least four servings of breads and cereals

A child's serving is not the same size as an adult's serving. A child's serving should be made up of one tablespoon for each year of the child's life. One serving of beans for a 6-year-old child would be 6 tablespoons.

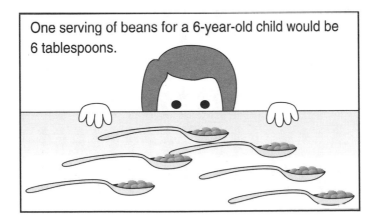

One serving of beans for a 6-year-old child would be 6 tablespoons.

This is just a guide. Children will eat more on some days than on others. Bigger children will eat more; smaller children will eat less.

Teenagers

Teens grow faster than anyone except infants. People put on about half of their adult weight during their teen years. Because of this, teens need a lot of calories.

Teens are often fond of such **"junk foods"** as chips, candy, cookies, and soda. These foods can provide the calories they need. But they provide empty calories. They will not provide the nutrients that teens need at the same time.

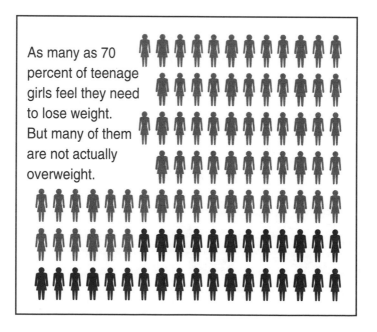

As many as 70 percent of teenage girls feel they need to lose weight. But many of them are not actually overweight.

Teenage girls often have more unbalanced diets than boys. As many as 70 percent of teenage girls feel they need to lose weight. But many of them are not actually overweight.

Many teenage girls go on harmful **weight-loss diets.** Such diets are short on the nutrients the teenager needs. Following these diets for a long time can harm a person's health.

Older adults

Many adults find that they gain weight as they get older. This can happen even if they eat the same as they did in their 20s. This happens for two reasons:

- Older people tend to be less active than younger people.
- As you get older your body loses muscle and gains fat. Fat uses fewer calories than muscle.

For these reasons, you do not need as many calories as you grow older. Of course, you can avoid these problems by staying active. If you become less active, you will need fewer calories.

Though you may need fewer calories, you still need the same amount of nutrients. So it is more important than ever to eat foods that are rich in nutrients.

Here is how your nutrient needs change as you get older:

- **Fiber.** Many older people have a hard time chewing foods that are full of fiber. Therefore, they sometimes do not eat enough fiber. This can lead to trouble having bowel movements. Because of this, many elderly people use **laxatives.** Laxatives can keep your body from absorbing some vitamins and minerals.

  It is better to use **stool softeners** than laxatives. Drinking a lot of water can help bowel movements. Regular physical activity also helps.

- **Sugar.** Older people's bodies cannot process sugar as well as younger people's. Older people should limit foods and drinks with sugar.

- **Fat and cholesterol.** Many older people believe it is too late to improve the health of their hearts by cutting down on fat and cholesterol. That is not true. A diet low in fat and cholesterol can help lower your risk of heart disease at any age.

Pregnant women

Good nutrition for a child begins while it is still in its mother's womb. Actually, it begins

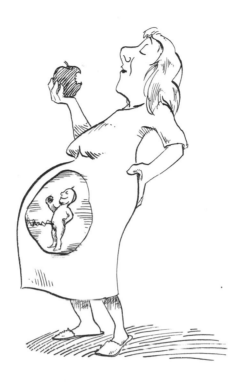

even before that. A woman who has a healthy diet is more likely to be able to get pregnant. She is also more likely to have a healthy baby.

Doctors used to tell women not to gain a lot of weight during pregnancy. Now we know that women who gain little or no weight during pregnancy are more likely to have very small babies. These babies tend to have more health problems than bigger babies. Now doctors say most women should gain from 24 to 35 pounds during pregnancy.

A pregnant woman needs to make healthy food choices. The baby she is carrying needs a lot of nutrients to grow well.

Chapter 4

Planning and Preparing

Plan your menu ahead of time. That way you can make sure you include all the nutrients you need. If you plan your menu for a whole week, you can get all your groceries in one trip.

Use the Food Guide Pyramid on page 35 to plan your meals. Try to include the suggested number of servings from each food group.

How much is in a serving? The chart on pages 50–51 gives serving sizes for the different food groups. Remember, for a child the serving size is smaller.

Serving Sizes

Type of food	How much is a serving?	Some examples
dairy products	• about 1 cup	• 1 cup yogurt • 1 cup milk • 1 egg • 1 1/2 slices of cheese • 1/2 cup cottage cheese
meat	• 2–3 ounces (oz.) of lean cooked meat	• steak • hamburger • chicken • fish • 1 egg
beans/ legumes	• 1 cup	• a bowl of chili • 1 cup of baked beans • a bowl of split-pea soup • 3-bean salad

Type of food	How much is a serving?	Some examples
fruits and vegetables	• 1/2 cup cooked or 1 cup raw • 1 piece of whole fruit or 1/2 cup of juice	• 1/2 cup of steamed broccoli • 1 raw shredded carrot • 1 banana • 1/2 cup of grapefruit juice • 1/4 cup of dried fruit • 1 apple
breads and grains	• 1 slice of bread • 1 cup of cold cereal • 3/4 cup of hot cereal • 1 cup of cooked pasta	• 1 piece of whole-wheat toast • 1 bowl of cereal • pasta with tomato sauce • 1 small muffin • 1/2 cup of cooked rice

A main meal, such as lunch or dinner, often includes five parts. They are:

- main dish
- bread, rice, or noodles
- vegetable or fruit
- milk, water, or other drink
- dessert

When planning, think about how much time you have to prepare meals. Also keep in mind how much money you can spend.

Compare your daily meal plan to the Food Guide Pyramid. Have you included the suggested number of servings from each food group?

If you have included less than the suggested total for a group, plan a snack from that group. You should think of a snack as part of your diet, not as something extra.

If you have included more than the suggested total servings, see where you can cut down. This is extra important if you have gone over on meats or fats.

Compare your menus for different days. Make sure you are not eating the same things each day. Remember, varying your menu helps you to get all the nutrients you need. It also makes your diet more interesting.

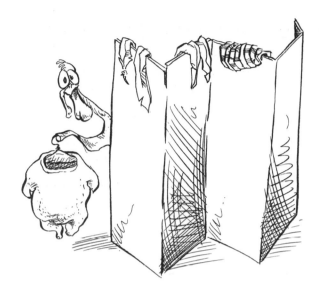

Preparing to Cut Down

If you are eating too much fat, see where you can cut down. Here are some things to try:

- Instead of frying, prepare food by baking, steaming, broiling, or roasting.
- Remove the skin from chicken or turkey before cooking.
- Cut the fat off meat before cooking.
- Use low-fat sprays instead of butter or oil to coat pans.
- Drink low-fat or skim milk rather than whole milk.

- Replace high-fat ingredients with low-fat ones. For example, use plain low-fat yogurt instead of sour cream; sherbet instead of ice cream; or part-skim mozzarella instead of regular mozzarella. In baking, use applesauce instead of oil.
- Replace high-fat desserts with low-fat ones. Angel food cake, frozen fruit bars, and low-fat frozen yogurt are low-fat desserts.

You should also limit the amount of salt, cholesterol, and sugar in your diet.

To cut down on salt you can:

- Add less salt when cooking vegetables or meat. If you cut it out a little at a time, you may not even notice.
- Use other spices. Try different things and see what you like.

To cut down on cholesterol you can:

- Use spreads with little or no cholesterol instead of butter.
- In cooking, use egg whites or an egg substitute instead of whole eggs. If you must use whole eggs, cut down on the number of yolks. Two egg whites can replace one whole egg in a recipe.

To cut down on sugar you can:

- Little by little, reduce the amount you put on cereal or in tea. After a while, you may not want it at all.
- Use less than called for in recipes. Most recipes will still taste fine if you use half or three-quarters of the sugar they call for.

To find out more

Do you have questions about your diet, or about certain foods? Call:

The American Dietetic Association

(800) 366-1655

This is a nutrition hotline.

Chapter 5

Shopping

Do you often spend more money at the grocery store than you can afford? Do you come home with items that you had not planned to buy? Do you wonder if the food you buy contains all the nutrients you need?

Here are some shopping tips. They will help you buy the foods you need for a healthy diet. They will also help you save money.

Before you shop

- Make a list. Plan your meals for at least a week. Then list everything you will need.

Try to buy all your food for the week in one trip. If you run to the store three or four times each week, you increase the chances of buying items you don't need.

- Check newspapers for sale items. If chicken is on sale, plan a meal around it. Do not buy junk food just because it is on sale.

- Use coupons. But do not buy something just because you have a coupon. If it fits in with your food plan, put it on the list.

  Even if you have a coupon, make sure you are getting the best deal. Sometimes the **store brand,** even without a coupon, is cheaper than a **name brand** with a coupon.

  If you have coupons for several brands of the same item, take all the coupons with you. If it is the same food, buy the cheapest one.

- Eat before you go. Do not shop when you are hungry. If you are hungry, you are more likely to buy items that are not on your list.

At the store

- Take the time to shop. If you are rushed, you may not make the best decisions.

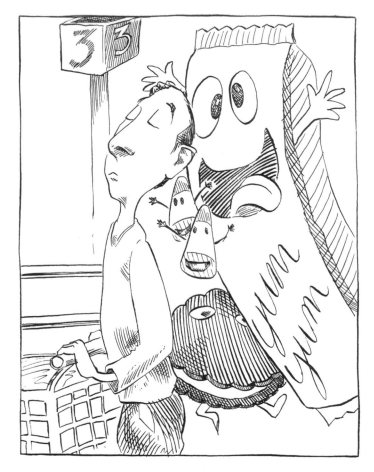

- Stick to your list. Ignore big displays at the ends of the aisles. Do the same with the candy at the checkout counter. They are put there to tempt you to buy things you do not need.
- Compare prices. Many stores have **unit pricing.** This shows how much each item

This box gives the unit price of the item. Compare the unit prices of different sizes and brands.

This box gives the price you'll pay for the item itself.

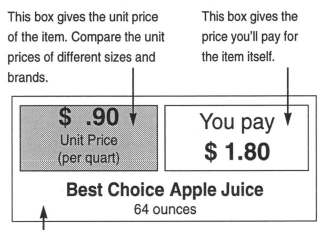

$ .90
Unit Price
(per quart)

You pay
$ 1.80

Best Choice Apple Juice
64 ounces

This area gives the name of the item and the amount in the package.

costs per ounce, per pound, or per quart. With unit prices, you can compare prices on items of different sizes.

- Read the labels. Under the law, most packaged foods have nutrition labels. Ingredient lists tell what is in the package. The list runs from the greatest to the least amount. For example, a cereal label might list sugar, then oats, then salt. That means the cereal contains more sugar than oats, and more oats than salt.

  The **nutrition facts box** lists the number of calories. This is the number of calories in each serving, not in the whole package.

It also lists the amounts of fat, protein, carbohydrate, and vitamins and minerals.

Many foods these days are labeled:

- light or "lite"
- diet
- sodium-free

These terms may be confusing. Sometimes they do not mean what you think. A "lite" food may have a lot of sodium. A "sodium-free" food may have a lot of fat.

Saving money at the grocery store

- Consider store brands or **white label (generic)** brands. They usually have the same nutrition content as name brands.
- Buy less tender cuts of meat. They are just as **nutritious.** You can tenderize them with a mallet, or use them in stews.
- Buy meat substitutes. Dried beans, peas, lentils, cheese, and eggs will give you the same nutrients as meat.
- Buy nonfat dry milk. You can use it for both cooking and drinking. If you do not like the taste, mix it half-and-half with regular low-fat milk.

Nutrition Facts

① Serving Size ½ cup (114g)
Servings Per Container 4

Amount Per Serving

② **Calories** 90   Calories from Fat 30

% Daily Value*

Total Fat 3g	**5%**
Saturated Fat 0g	**0%**
Cholesterol 0mg	**0%**
Sodium 300mg	**13%**
Total Carbohydrate 13g	**4%**
Dietary Fiber 3g	**12%**
Sugars 3g	
Protein 3g	

③

④

Vitamin A	80%	•	Vitamin C	60%
Calcium	4%	•	Iron	4%

* Percent Daily Values are based on a 2,000 calorie diet. Your daily values may be higher or lower depending on your calorie needs:

	Calories	2,000	2,500
Total Fat	Less than	65g	80g
Sat Fat	Less than	20g	25g
Cholesterol	Less than	300mg	300mg
Sodium	Less than	2,400mg	2,400mg
Total Carbohydrate		300g	375g
Fiber		25g	30g

Calories per gram:
Fat 9   •   Carbohydrate 4   •   Protein 4

Look for this new food label on packaged foods. It can help you make good food choices.

① **Serving size** shows a realistic amount of the food. Similar types of food have similar serving sizes.

② **Calories from fat** can help you decide if a food has too much fat.

③ **List of nutrients** can help you decide if a food has too much or too little of a certain nutrient.

④ **% Daily Value** shows how the food fits into your overall daily diet.

- Buy fewer prepared foods. It does take less time to heat up a microwave dinner or stew from a can. But making meals from scratch is cheaper.

Some of these tips can help you spend less for a balanced diet. By reading the label, you can compare nutrients in different foods. Reading labels also helps you limit the fat and sodium you eat.

Staying away from highly **processed foods** helps, too. Foods may lose nutrients as they are processed. Also, prepared or processed foods often have a lot of added salt or sugar.

Another way to make sure you are getting all your nutrients is to vary what you buy each week. Try a new fruit or vegetable. Buy rye or wheat bread instead of white. Try out some new recipes. This is a good way to keep your diet interesting, too.

Other Places to Buy Your Food

You do not need to get all your food at a supermarket. You might want to get some of it at a farmers' market or through a food co-op.

Farmers' markets

Many cities and towns have farmers' markets. Most run once or twice a week.

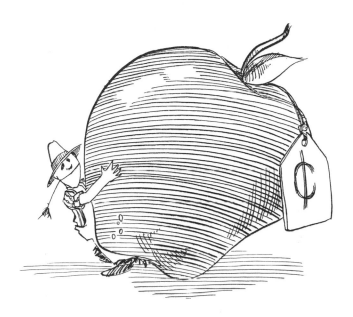

Farmers bring their fruits and vegetables to these markets. Because the farmers are selling their own produce, the prices are usually lower than in supermarkets. The fruits and vegetables are usually very fresh.

Food co-ops

In some communities, people join together in food co-ops. They buy foods in large quantities. This makes them cheaper.

If there is a food co-op nearby, you may want to consider joining it. First, though, look at which foods they buy for their members. Are these foods that you use?

There is another cost at a food co-op—your time. Members are expected to put in some time working at the co-op. This is one way that co-ops are able to keep prices low.

To find out more

For more information about saving money and shopping smart, look for pamphlets at your local supermarket.

You can also call your local agricultural (or "cooperative") extension service. Look in your phone book for the number.

Chapter 6
Handling Food

Each year, about two million people in the U.S. get **food poisoning.** Most of them get nothing more serious than an upset stomach. Many victims think they have the flu.

Most cases of food poisoning clear up by themselves. Sometimes, however, food poisoning can cause serious illness. Some people die from it.

Food goes bad because of **bacteria.** They are often too tiny to see. They get into food and grow. Some **spoiled food** looks or smells bad. If a food in your refrigerator smells or looks bad, throw it out. Do not taste it.

Sometimes you are not sure whether food has gone bad. It may smell just a little funny. Do not taste it. Just throw it out. It is better to waste the food than to get ill.

Some spoiled food looks and smells all right. It may taste OK, too. But it is full of food-poisoning bacteria. How do you keep from eating such food? The best way is to keep the bacteria from growing in the first place.

There are two things you can do to prevent food poisoning:

- buy safe food
- keep it safe at home

Buying safe food

- Buy cans and jars that look perfect. Cans should not bulge or have dents. Jars should not be cracked. Their lids should be closed tight.
- Check eggs for cracks.
- Choose food that looks fresh. If meat or produce looks old, choose something else.
- Keep uncooked meat juices away from other food. You can put meat, **poultry,** and

seafood into plastic bags before you put them in your cart.

- Check **"sell by" dates** on containers. If the date is already past, do not buy the food.

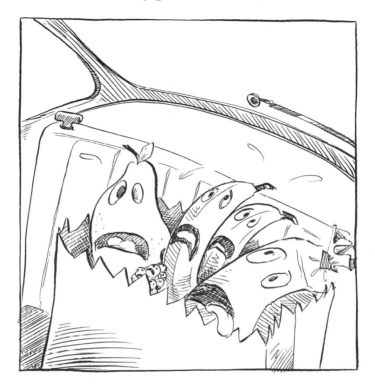

- Pick up milk and other cold foods last. This gives them less time to warm up on the way home. Go right home after shopping. Do not leave food in the car while you run errands.

Keeping food safe at home

- Put food away as soon as you get it home.
- Wash your hands before and after you handle food. Also, wash your hands when you have finished handling one food, and before you handle another. Use warm water and soap.
- Make sure the kitchen is clean. Wash counters before and after you prepare food on them.
- Make sure your dishes and utensils are clean. Wash dishes and utensils before and after they touch food.
- Wash kitchen cloths often. If you use a cloth to wipe up juice from meat, poultry, or seafood, put it right in the laundry. Or use paper towels and throw them away.
- Rinse raw fruits and vegetables under running water.
- Keep raw meat, poultry, and seafood away from other foods.
- Thaw meat, poultry, and seafood in the refrigerator. Or defrost them in a microwave. Then cook them right away. Do not thaw meats on the kitchen counter.
- Make sure foods are cooked all the way through. Chicken juices should be clear,

not pink. Fish should be flaky. Egg whites and yolks should be firm, not runny.

- Keep hot foods hot and cold foods cold. Put leftovers in the refrigerator right away. Food should not be left out of the refrigerator or off the stove for more than two hours. These two hours include *all time* that the food has not been in the oven, on the stove, or in the refrigerator.
- Check **"use by" dates** on containers. If the date is past, throw the food out.

Storing Food

It's important to store foods in the right place and not to keep them for too long. Here are some general guidelines for storing food.

Dairy products

Store all dairy products in the refrigerator. Check the "use by" date on the following foods. Throw them away once the date is past.

- milk
- cream
- cheese
- yogurt
- eggs

Meats

Most meats can be stored in the refrigerator or freezer. Red meat can stay in the refrigerator for three to five days. It should be frozen if it won't be used in that time. Uncooked red meat can be frozen for three to six months.

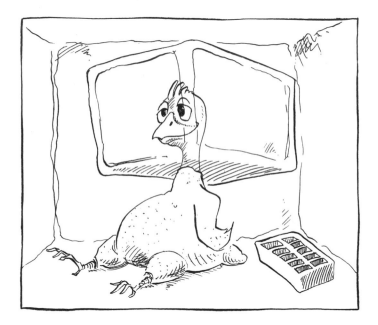

Chicken

Chicken should only stay in the refrigerator for one to two days. If you're not going to use it that soon, put chicken in the freezer. It can stay there for nine months to a year.

To find out more

For more information on storage times and how to keep your food safe, call:

USDA Meat and Poultry Hotline

(800) 535-4555

You can also call your local agricultural (or "cooperative") extension service. Look in your phone book for the number.

Chapter 7
Eating Out

Eating out is a big part of many people's diet. In the U.S., adults get as much as 30 percent of their calories away from home.

Think of meals eaten out as part of your whole diet. You may feel that you cannot control what you eat when you are out. But you do decide where to eat and what to order.

Here are some tips to make eating out fit in with the rest of your diet:

- Carefully choose where you will eat. This affects the food choices that you will have.

Sit-down restaurants usually have the biggest menus. Food is most often prepared to order. You can ask that a dish be prepared in a different way than on the menu. For example, ask for grilled chicken instead of fried.

Cafeterias and buffets also offer a lot of choices. The food is already prepared, though. You are not able to order foods a special way.

Fast-food restaurants offer limited menus. Many items are deep-fat fried. In recent years, though, they have started to expand their menus. Most offer salads. Some have baked potatoes and whole-grain rolls. Some will cook certain items to order.

• Make healthy food choices. Follow the same rules that guide your choices when eating at home.

If you choose to eat food that is high in fat, salt, or cholesterol, stick to a small portion.

Do not be afraid to ask for what you want. Remember, you are paying. Restaurants cannot handle every request, but many will do their best.

If you sometimes choose a meal high in fat, cholesterol, or sodium, it is not the end of the world. Everyone splurges once in a while.

Useful clues

Certain words on the menu can give you a clue about fat and sodium content. A dish is usually high in fat if it is described as:

- buttered
- fried
- breaded
- creamed
- hollandaise
- with gravy
- au gratin
- scalloped
- rich
- pastry

A dish probably has a lot of sodium if it is described as:

- smoked
- pickled
- barbecued
- in broth
- in cocktail sauce
- in a tomato base

- with soy sauce
- teriyaki
- creole sauce
- mustard sauce
- marinated
- Parmesan

Chapter 8

Weight Control

How much a person should weigh to be healthy varies from person to person. Check with a doctor to see if your weight is healthy.

There are many reasons why people become overweight. Some people fall into unhealthy eating habits. Others cut back on exercise without cutting back on the amount of food they eat. Some people eat too much when they are anxious or upset.

Some people are overweight but don't eat too much. These people may have a family history of weight problems. Or they may have a medical condition.

Being overweight is unhealthy. It increases your chances of getting heart disease, diabetes, high blood pressure, and even cancer.

Some fat people feel bad about themselves. They may think they are too weak-willed to lose weight and keep it off. This is not true. Willpower has little to do with keeping weight off. What is important is learning good eating and exercise habits.

Dieting

You can lose weight by dieting, so long as you change your eating habits. Healthy eating habits help you maintain a healthy weight.

Many people become "yo-yo" dieters. They lose weight and regain it. They do this again and again. They never manage to keep the weight off.

Yo-yo dieting puts a lot of strain on your heart. Sometimes it is better just to stay overweight. Check with your doctor to find out what is best for you. To avoid yo-yo dieting, you must plan to change eating and exercise habits for life.

Many weight-loss diets do not teach people how to change their eating habits forever. Most

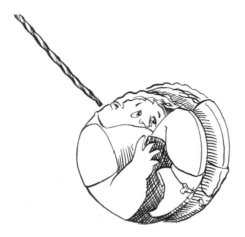

people think of dieting as something you do just for a while.

Some weight-loss diets are not based on good nutrition. Many of them fail to provide all the nutrients you need to stay healthy. Some are even dangerous.

There is an answer, though. You can lose weight and keep it off. You do not need to diet. You need to teach yourself how to eat in a healthy way. You need to start exercising regularly.

Here are some steps to lose weight and keep it off:

- Forget about losing weight quickly. It took years to put on those extra pounds. It will take time to get rid of them.

- Keep a food diary. Write down everything you eat or drink. Write down the amount. Write down when you ate, and where. Also write down why you ate. Were you hungry, or were you just bored? Keep this diary for a couple of weeks.

  It may surprise you to see how much you really eat. You may begin to see what causes you to eat when you are not hungry. Some people eat when they are upset or bored. Other people overeat at certain times of day.

- Begin to change your unhealthy habits. Do this slowly. Make small changes at first. For example, you might want to replace your high-calorie afternoon snack. Try cut-up vegetables and a low-calorie dip, or fruit. After you have changed one habit, move on to another.

- Let your body tell you when it needs food. Do not eat unless you are hungry. Your body tells you when it needs food.

- Eat what you like. Do not forbid yourself certain foods. This will just make you want them more. If your favorite foods are high in fat or calories, eat them less often and in small amounts.

- Exercise. This will increase the number of calories your body uses. It will also build muscle. The more muscle you have, the better your body uses calories.

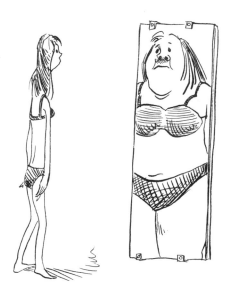

When You Cannot Stop Dieting

Some people cannot stop dieting. They see themselves as fat, no matter how thin they get. They eat little or no food. These people may have anorexia.

There is another eating disease, called bulimia. Its victims binge. That means they eat huge amounts of food. Then they vomit to get rid of the calories.

Both diseases happen mostly to teenage girls. Other people can get them, though. Anorexia and bulimia are very dangerous. Some people starve themselves to death. Others harm their health forever. Anyone who has one of these diseases should see a doctor right away.

Chapter 9
Conclusion

Life Stories, Continued

Remember the life stories back in the beginning of the book? Those people all needed to improve their diets. Here's what they have learned from this book.

Andrea and Mike

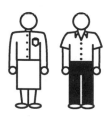 Andrea and Mike are the married couple. They do not like to cook. They do not have a lot of time for it, either.

The couple used to have donuts and coffee for breakfast. They still drink coffee. They have replaced the donuts, though. Donuts have a lot of fat. That was not helping Mike's weight and cholesterol problems.

Andrea and Mike have come up with some low-fat choices for breakfast. They sometimes have low-fat cereal with skim milk. Other times they have toast, English muffins, or bagels with low-calorie spread and a glass of skim milk. These choices are quick to prepare.

The next problem area was lunch. Andrea eats in the cafeteria at work. Usually she has a sandwich or a salad. These are not bad choices. She is more careful now about how they are prepared, though.

If Andrea has a sandwich, she asks for it on whole-grain bread. Instead of mayonnaise, she often has mustard, which is lower in fat.

When she orders a salad, she asks for dressing on the side. She uses the dressing as a dip. This way, she does not eat as much of it. She also buys a whole-grain roll.

Mike used to skip lunch or eat a hot dog or grilled cheese sandwich. Now, he makes sure to eat lunch every day. This keeps him from grabbing chips or candy in the afternoon.

Mike buys his lunch from the truck that comes to his work site. The choices are limited, but he can get a turkey or tuna sandwich. This cuts down on the fat he was getting from the hot dog or grilled cheese.

Instead of the soda he used to drink with lunch, Mike now buys skim or 2% milk.

Both Andrea and Mike have gotten into the habit of taking fruit, cut-up vegetables, or low-fat yogurt to work with them. They eat them for snacks or with their lunches.

Dinner was the biggest problem for Andrea and Mike. They get home late. They eat canned soups, frozen dinners, and take-out food.

The first thing they did was to start reading labels at the store. Now they buy soups and frozen dinners with less fat and sodium.

Andrea and Mike still eat a lot of take-out food. But they are more careful about what they buy. They stay away from fatty items such as fried rice and french fries. They order lower-fat

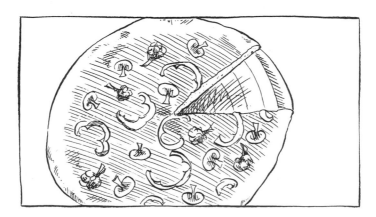

foods like pizza with vegetable toppings instead of extra cheese.

Andrea and Mike have even started to cook some. On the weekends, they make casseroles. They eat one portion when they make it. They freeze the rest. They also make a point of getting exercise every weekend.

When they get home from work they can thaw the frozen dinner in the microwave. It is already cooked. It just needs to be heated up.

Andrea knows she will need to keep up these good habits if she gets pregnant. Good eating habits will help her baby grow healthy.

Sonya

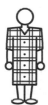 Sonya is the single mother. Her kids each love different foods. They all love sugar, though. One daughter has a problem with tooth decay. She should not have so much sugar.

Sonya is also worried about money. Each week, she spends more money than she plans to on food.

The first thing Sonya did was to change her shopping habits. She used to take the girls with her. They nagged her for all the sugary foods they love. After a while, Sonya would get tired of arguing. She would give in. She would rush through the shopping just to get it over with.

Now, Sonya leaves the girls with a neighbor when she goes shopping. Then she watches the neighbor's children while he shops.

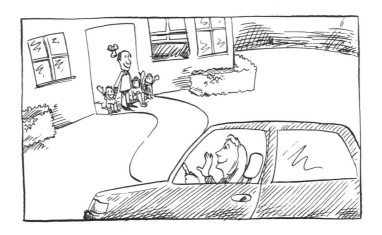

Now that she shops alone, Sonya can take her time. She can compare prices. She can read the labels. Without her daughters there begging, she buys fewer sugary foods.

Just by shopping carefully, Sonya saves about $15 each week. On weeks when her neighbor cannot watch the girls, she hires a baby-sitter. Even after paying the baby-sitter, she still saves money.

The second thing Sonya changed was her thinking about mealtimes. She used to dread meals. She spent most of her time trying to get the girls to eat. They spent most of their time resisting. Now Sonya worries less about getting her daughters to eat. None of them is too thin. They must be getting enough calories. Meals are not so tense anymore.

Sonya has also changed her menus. She does not give in to the girls' desire for sugary junk food. She fixes a healthy main dish. She also offers a few choices with the meals, such as cut-up fruit and vegetables.

The girls do not like everything Sonya serves. They have started to try a few new things, though. Since they have a few choices, they can usually find something they like at each meal. Also, since they don't eat the sweets, they are hungrier for the real food.

Karl

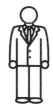 Karl has high blood pressure. His doctor said he should lose weight and cut most of the sodium out of his diet. He knew he needed to change, but he loved his fatty, high-sodium diet.

Because of his job, Karl eats out a lot. The first thing he changed was where he ate. He tries now to choose sit-down restaurants when he can. At these restaurants, the menus offer more choices.

Karl has started ordering broiled or baked meat. He has started cutting down on the salt he used to shake onto almost everything.

Karl hated making these changes at first. Soon, though, he found out he liked broiled and baked dishes. After a while, he stopped putting salt on his food. He realized he had been tasting mainly the salt, not the food. Now he dislikes the taste of salted food.

Karl has started ordering a salad and a whole-grain roll with his dinner. Now, when it comes time for dessert, he often finds he is full. If he does want dessert, he orders a small portion, or shares it.

Karl has made changes at home, too. He used to eat many canned fruits and vegetables. He thought they were easier to prepare. He has started buying fresh fruits and vegetables instead. He found out that most of them need little or no preparation. He can just steam them, or eat them raw.

At snack times, Karl has stopped reaching for cookies and cake. Raw fruits and vegetables are a better choice. All he has to do is wash or peel them, and they're ready to eat.

Karl broils meat at home now. He's surprised at how easy it is. He has not yet broken the habit of putting butter on bread and

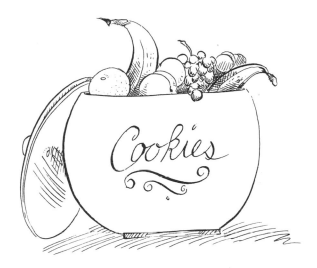

vegetables. But he has cut down on the amount he uses.

Karl did not think he had made major changes in his diet. But when he went for his next checkup, he was surprised. He had lost five pounds in six weeks. His blood pressure is starting to go down.

He still has a long way to go, but he feels good. He knows he has changed his diet forever.

The people in the life stories are using the guidelines set out at the beginning of the book:

- Eat many kinds of foods.
- Do not eat too much of any one food.
- Change your eating habits slowly.

Andrea and Mike, Sonya and her daughters, and Karl don't have perfect diets. But they have learned to make better food choices. They have learned that even small changes can make you healthier.

In the future, these people may make more changes in the way they eat. They now know that eating healthy does not have to be hard. They know they do not have to give up the foods they love. They know good nutrition does not have to cost a lot of money.

Andrea and Mike, Sonya, and Karl have learned that eating right will help them to stay healthy. If they do get sick, good eating habits will help them to get well more quickly. Adding exercise has helped Andrea and Mike stay healthy, too.

They also know that eating a healthy diet makes them feel good. It gives them the energy they need for all the things they want to do in life.

Glossary

addicted: having a strong physical need for a habit-forming drug

anemia: lack of iron in the blood. Anemia causes weakness and paleness.

bacteria: tiny organisms that cause diseases. They also cause food to go bad.

calories: units measuring the energy provided by food

cholesterol: a substance in animal fat that can build up inside the body and cause heart disease

diabetes: a disease that means people have too much sugar in their blood. Diabetes can cause many health problems.

dietary fiber: the fiber in food

digest: turning food into substances the body can use

fiber: a substance that helps the body get rid of waste and that keeps the digestive system strong

Food Guide Pyramid: a chart that shows how much of each type of food people need to eat every day

food poisoning: illness caused by eating spoiled food. Signs of food poisoning include stomach cramps, vomiting, diarrhea, and fever. Severe food poisoning can cause death.

heart disease: weakening of the heart that can lead to chest pain, heart attack, or stroke. It is also called *cardiovascular disease.*

high blood pressure: a disease that can lead to heart disease and other health problems. It is also called *hypertension.*

infant formula: food for babies that contains many of the nutrients found in breast milk

ingredient list: the list on packaged food or drink that says exactly what the food or drink contains

junk foods: foods that are high in empty calories but low in nutrients. Most junk foods contain a lot of fat, sugar, or sodium.

laxatives: medicines that help make the bowels loose and relieve constipation

multivitamin: a pill that includes many different vitamins and minerals. A person doesn't need a prescription to get them.

name brand: a brand that is made by one company and sold in many different stores

nutrients: the useful materials the body gets from food

nutrition: food or drink and what the body gets from it

nutrition facts box: the list on packaged food or drink that says exactly what nutrients are in the food or drink. It usually tells how much a person needs of each nutrient every day, and how much one serving of the food or drink provides.

nutritionist: a food expert who studies what food the body needs and how to get it

nutritious: providing nutrients

osteoporosis: a disease that causes brittle bones

poultry: chicken, turkey, duck, goose, and other fowl

processed foods: foods that have been treated in some way. Most foods in cans and jars are processed.

saturated fat: the worst kind of fat for the body. It builds up, sometimes leading to heart disease. Saturated fats are in animal products—meat, whole milk, cheese, eggs, butter, etc.

"sell by" date: a date stamped on many packages of food in the store. The food is too old to sell after that date.

sodium: an element in salt. Too much sodium leads to high blood pressure and other health problems.

soy milk: a kind of milk made from soy beans

spoiled food: food that contains harmful bacteria. Food can spoil two hours after it is taken out of the refrigerator or oven.

stool softeners: products, including bran, that make the stool soft and so help bowel movements

store brand: a brand that has the name of the store or another special name on it. Safeway and A & P are store brands.

stroke: an attack during which blood doesn't flow freely to the brain. It can cause brain damage, paralysis, and even death.

tissues: the solid parts of the body (for example, bones, muscles, fat)

tooth decay: the action of certain bacteria leading to cavities. Many foods help the bacteria to multiply, but sugars are the worst.

unit pricing: signs on grocery store shelves that let customers compare prices of different packages of food. They tell how much each food costs per unit (for example, per pound or per pint).

unsaturated fat: fat that does not build up cholesterol in your body. Olive oil and most nut oils are unsaturated fats.

"use by" date: the date stamped on many
packages of food. The food is too old to use
after that date.

vegetarians: people who don't eat meat. Some
vegetarians don't eat dairy products or eggs.

weight-loss diet: a special diet with a goal of
losing weight

white label (generic): packages of food that do
not have brand names or store names on
them. They are usually the cheapest of all.
They usually have white labels with black
print.

yo-yo dieting: repeated weight-loss dieting
followed by gaining weight again. The body
weight goes up and down all the time.